# PREGNANCY COOKBOOK

## MAIN COURSE - 60+ Breakfast, Lunch, Dinner and Dessert Recipes to support your health during and after pregnancy

# TABLE OF CONTENTS

purposes solely, and is universal as so. The presentation of the information is without contract or any type of guarantee assurance.

The trademarks that are used are without any consent, and the publication of the trademark is without permission or backing by the trademark owner. All trademarks and brands within this book are for clarifying purposes only and are the owned by the owners themselves, not affiliated with this document.

Introduction

Pregnancy recipes for personal enjoyment but also for family enjoyment. You will love them for sure for how easy it is to prepare them.

## FRENCH TOAST

Serves:          **2**
Prep Time:     **5**     minutes

Cook Time:     **5**     minutes

Total Time:    **10**    minutes

### INGREDIENTS

- 1 ½ tsp cinnamon
- 4 slices bread
- 2 tsp vanilla
- 4 eggs
- 3 tbs milk

### DIRECTIONS

1. Whisk together the eggs, milk, vanilla and cinnamon in a bowl
2. Soak the bread into the mixture
3. Heat a greased pan

4. Cook the soaked bread for about 2 minutes per side until golden
5. Serve immediately

Serves:          **4**

Prep Time:    **10**   Minutes

Cook Time:   **15**   Minutes

Total Time:   **25**   Minutes

## INGREDIENTS

- 1 cup quinoa
- 2 tbs almonds
- 3 tbs coconut
- 1/3 tsp cinnamon
- 1 cup strawberries
- 2 cups milk
- 3 tbs maple syrup

## DIRECTIONS

1. Place the quinoa and the milk in a pot and bring to a boil
2. Reduce the heat and simmer for at least 10 minutes

3. Stir in 2 extra tbs of milk, maple syrup and cinnamon

4. Divide into bowls and top with strawberries, coconut and almonds

Serves: *1*

Prep Time: 5 Minutes

Cook Time: 5 Minutes

Total Time: *10* Minutes

## INGREDIENTS

- 4 slices tomato
- 1 oz cheese
- 2 tbs mayonnaise
- 1 slice bread
- 1 can sardines
- ¼ tsp turmeric
- A pinch salt
- A pinch black pepper

## DIRECTIONS

1. Mix the sardines, mayonnaise, turmeric and salt
2. Toast the bread
3. Spread the mixture over the bread

4. Top with tomato slices and then with the cheese slices

5. Broil in the preheated oven for 2 minutes

6. Serve topped with black pepper

Serves:         2

Prep Time:   5   Minutes

Cook Time:   5   Minutes

Total Time:  10  Minutes

## INGREDIENTS

- 2 cups coconut milk
- Raspberries
- 1 banana
- ½ cup rolled oats
- Handful spinach leaves
- 1/3 cup chia seeds
- ½ mango
- 1 pear

## DIRECTIONS

1. Place the banana, spinach and coconut milk in a food processor and pulse until smooth
2. Stir in the chia seeds and the oats, mixing well

3. Refrigerate covered overnight
4. Peel and dice the mango
5. Top the oats with mango, pear and raspberries
6. Serve when ready

Serves: **2**

Prep Time: **5** Minutes

Cook Time: **5** Minutes

Total Time: **10** Minutes

## INGREDIENTS

- 1/3 cup black beans
- 3 tbs salsa
- 1 scallion
- 2 tbs cilantro
- 2 eggs
- 1 tortilla
- ½ avocado
- 1 tomato
- 1/3 cup shredded cheese

## DIRECTIONS

1. Cook the salsa, black beans, cilantro and scallions for about 2 minutes

2. Add in the eggs and cook until set
3. Heat the tortilla
4. Spoon the cooked mixture onto the tortilla, then top with diced avocado, tomato and cheese
5. Roll-up the tortilla and cut in half
6. Serve immediately

Serves:        *12*
Prep Time:    *10*    Minutes

Cook Time:    *50*    Minutes

Total Time:   *60*    Minutes

## INGREDIENTS

- 2 bananas
- 2 eggs
- 3 tsp vanilla
- 1 cup flour
- 1 tsp cinnamon
- ½ tsp nutmeg
- 1 cup grape juice
- 1 tsp baking soda
- 1/3 cup walnuts
- ¼ cup oil
- 2 tbs baking powder
- 1/3 cup oat bran
- 1/3 cup oats

## DIRECTIONS

1. Mix the banana, oil, eggs, vanilla and eggs in a blender and pulse until smooth

2. Mix the flaxseed, oats, flour, nutmeg, cinnamon, baking soda and baking powder in a separate bowl and stir well

3. Stir in the banana mixture into the flour mixture, mixing gently

4. Fold in the walnuts

5. Spoon the batter into a greased pan

6. Cook in the preheated oven for 50 minutes at 350F

7. Allow to cool, then serve

Serves:         *4*
Prep Time:   *10*  Minutes

Cook Time:  *10*  Minutes

Total Time:  *20*  Minutes

## INGREDIENTS

- 2 cup blueberries
- 2 tsp baking powder
- 1 ½ cup flour
- 2 tsp baking soda
- 2 eggs
- 1/3 cup oil
- 1/3 cup grape juice
- 1/3 tsp vanilla
- 1/3 cup oats
- 1 ½ cups buttermilk

## DIRECTIONS

1. Mix together the flour, baking powder and baking soda and the oats

2. Whisk the eggs with ¼ cup oil, grape juice and vanilla in a separate bowl

3. Pour the buttermilk and the egg mixture over the dry ingredients

4. Stir to combine, then fold in the blueberries

5. Cook the pancakes in 1 tbs of hot oil

6. Cook on both sides until golden brown

7. Serve topped with maple syrup

Serves: **8**

Prep Time: **10** Minutes

Cook Time: **20** Minutes

Total Time: **30** Minutes

## INGREDIENTS

- 4 oz butter
- 1 oz sesame seeds
- 1 oz flaxseeds
- 2 oz nuts
- 3 oz rolled oats
- 1 egg
- 3 oz
- 4 oz dates
- 3 tbs syrup

## DIRECTIONS

1. Mix the butter and the syrup together
2. Beat the eggs and mix with the almonds

3. Stir in the egg mixture into the butter mixture
4. Mix in the remaining ingredients
5. Pour into a greased baking tin and bake for at least 20 minutes
6. Allow to cool, then serve

Serves:        2
Prep Time:    5    Minutes

Cook Time:  10   Minutes

Total Time:  15   Minutes


## INGREDIENTS

- Grated apple
- 1 tsp flaxseed
- Handful sultanas
- 1 ½ tsp maca
- Apple puree
- Nuts
- Honey
- Handful cranberries
- 1 banana
- 1 dollop yogurt
- Blueberries
- Raspberries

## DIRECTIONS

1. Prepare the porridge as you desire
2. Stir in the remaining ingredients
3. Cook over gentle heat until thick
4. Serve immediately

Serves:        **2**
Prep Time:   **10**   Minutes

Cook Time:   **20**   Minutes

Total Time:   **30**   Minutes

## INGREDIENTS

- 1/3 cup sunflower, pumpkin, sesame and chia seeds
- 1 cup pecan nuts
- 2 cups rolled oats
- 1/3 cup cranberries
- 1/3 cup almonds
- 1/3 cup coconut oil
- 1/3 cup peanut butter
- 1/3 cup water
- ½ cup honey

## DIRECTIONS

1. **Mix the dry ingredients together**

2. Mix the coconut oil, honey, water and peanut butter together in a bowl

3. Mix in the wet ingredients into the dry ingredients until combined

4. Pour the mixture into a lined baking sheet

5. Bake in the preheated oven at 350F for at least 15 minutes

6. Allow to cool, then serve

## HUMMUS PITA

Serves: **1**

Prep Time: **5** Minutes

Cook Time: **10** Minutes

Total Time: **15** Minutes

### INGREDIENTS

- ½ cup spinach
- 1 ½ tbs pine nuts
- ¼ cup hummus
- 2 eggs
- ¼ cup tomato
- 1 pita

### DIRECTIONS

1. Boil the eggs until hard
2. Cut the pita in half
3. Fill both halves with the remaining ingredients

4. Serve immediately

Serves:          **6**
Prep Time:    **10**   Minutes

Cook Time:    **60**   Minutes

Total Time:   **70**   Minutes

## INGREDIENTS

- 1 tsp thyme
- 15 oz chicken broth
- ½ cup apple juice
- 1 ½ tbs olive oil
- 1 celery stalk
- 1 cup parmesan
- 2 leeks
- 2 carrots
- 2 lb butternut squash
- Salt
- Pepper

## DIRECTIONS

1. Cut the squash and drizzle with oil, then season with salt and pepper
2. Bake in the preheated oven at 350 F for at least 50 minutes
3. Cook the leeks, carrots and celery for 15 minutes in hot oil until softened
4. Scrape squash into processor and discard peel
5. Pour in 1 cup of broth and puree until smooth
6. Mix in apple juice and season with salt and pepper
7. Garnish each bowl with parmesan cheese and serve

Serves:      **2**

Prep Time:   **10**  Minutes

Cook Time:  **10**  Minutes

Total Time:  **20**  Minutes

## INGREDIENTS

- 1 onion
- 2 cloves garlic
- 1 tbs butter
- 2 cup broccoli
- 1 potato
- 3 cup chicken broth
- 1 cup cheddar cheese
- 1/3 cup buttermilk
- Salt
- Pepper

## DIRECTIONS

1. **Cook the onion and garlic in melted butter for 5 minutes**

2. Add the diced potato, broccoli florets and chicken broth

3. Bring to a boil, then reduce the heat and simmer for at least 5 minutes

4. Allow to cool, then pulse until smooth using a blender

5. Return to the saucepan and add the buttermilk and ¼ cup cheese

6. Cook for about 3 minutes

7. Season with salt and pepper

8. Serve topped with the remaining cheese

Serves:        **6**
Prep Time:    **40**   Minutes

Cook Time:    **80**   Minutes

Total Time:   **120**  Minutes

## INGREDIENTS

**Broth:**
- 15 peppercorns
- 2 onions
- 2 carrots
- 1 rib celery
- 3 sprigs thyme
- 5 cloves garlic
- 3 bay leaves
- 8 chicken thighs

**Soup:**
- 2 chicken bouillon cubes
- 1 tsp salt
- 5 oz egg noodles
- 1/3 cup parsley

- 2 ribs celery
- 2 carrots

## DIRECTIONS

1. Place the broth ingredients in a pot with 12 cups of water
2. Bring to a boil, then reduce the heat and simmer for about 20 minutes
3. Remove the chicken and shred meat from bones
4. Return the bones to the pot and continue to simmer for another 60 minutes
5. Strain the broth and discard the bones and other solids
6. Skim broth and bring to a boil
7. Add the soup ingredients except for the parsley
8. Stir in the noodles and cook for at least 5 minutes
9. Stir in the chicken meat and parsley and cook 1 more minute
10. Serve immediately

Serves:         **6**
Prep Time:   **10**   Minutes

Cook Time:   **10**   Minutes

Total Time:   **20**   Minutes

## INGREDIENTS

- 1/3 cup rice
- 15 oz salsa
- 1 can black beans
- 30 oz chicken broth
- 1 cup corn
- Chicken

## DIRECTIONS

1. **Place the broth and the salsa in a pot and bring to a boil**
2. **Add rice, beans and cooked chicken**
3. **Simmer covered for about 10 minutes**
4. **Stir in the corn**

5. Serve topped with cheese

Serves:        *4*
Prep Time:    *15*  Minutes

Cook Time:    *35*  Minutes

Total Time:   *50*  Minutes

## INGREDIENTS

- 2 tbs oil
- 1/3 tsp salt
- 1 cup bread cubes
- 1 cup potato
- 2 tsp horseradish
- 3 cups chicken broth
- 1 lb asparagus
- Scallions
- 1 shallot

## DIRECTIONS

1. Cook the shallot until soft for 2 minutes

2. Add the asparagus, potato, broth, horseradish and salt and bring to a boil
3. Reduce the heat and simmer for about 15 minutes
4. Pulse using a blender
5. Cook the bread cubes in hot oil until crispy
6. Serve topped with croutons

Serves:         **9**
Prep Time:   **10**   Minutes

Cook Time:   **50**   Minutes

Total Time:   **60**   Minutes

## INGREDIENTS

- 2 tbs oil
- 1 stalk celery
- 1 red bell pepper
- 2 cans chicken broth
- 1 onion
- 1 cup carrots
- 2 garlic cloves
- 2 tsp cumin
- 1 tsp coriander
- 1 can tomatoes
- 2 sweet potatoes
- 3 tsp thyme leaves
- 2 cups red lentils

## DIRECTIONS

1. Cook the onion, celery, carrots and red pepper in hot oil for 3 minutes

2. Add garlic, thyme, cumin and coriander and cook for 10 more minutes

3. Add the broth, sweet potatoes, lentils and tomatoes

4. Bring to a boil, then reduce the heat and simmer for at least 30 minutes

5. Pulse using a blender

6. Serve immediately

Serves:           **1**

Prep Time:     **5**    Minutes

Cook Time:    **5**    Minutes

Total Time:    **10**   Minutes

## INGREDIENTS

- 1 cup rice
- ½ cup roasted red peppers
- ½ cup black beans
- ½ cup shrimp
- 3 tbs salsa
- ½ avocado

## DIRECTIONS

1. Cook the rice and the shrimp as you desire
2. Mix everything together
3. Serve topped with avocado slices

Serves:          *1*
Prep Time:   *10*   Minutes

Cook Time:   *10*   Minutes

Total Time:   *20*   Minutes

## INGREDIENTS

- ½ cup ground turkey
- 1 hatch chile
- Salt
- Pepper
- 1 cup spinach
- 1 tomato
- 1 onion
- ½ avocado

## DIRECTIONS

1. Mix the turkey meat with chiles, salt and pepper and forma patty
2. Grill until done

3. Serve on a bed of cooked spinach and top with tomatoes, onion and avocado slices

4. Serve immediately

Serves:         2
Prep Time:    5    Minutes

Cook Time:   10   Minutes

Total Time:   15   Minutes

## INGREDIENTS

- ½ cup spinach
- 1 tbs basil
- 2 cloves garlic
- 1 onion
- ½ cup sun dried tomatoes
- 2 roasted peppers
- ½ cup chicken breast
- 1 wheat naan
- ½ cup mozzarella

## DIRECTIONS

1. Top the naan with all of the ingredients
2. Bake for 10 minutes

**3. Serve immediately**

Serves:        2
Prep Time:    5    Minutes
Cook Time:    5    Minutes
Total Time:  *10*   Minutes

## INGREDIENTS

- 1 can unsweetened pineapple
- 1 package cherry gelatin
- 1 tablespoon lemon juice
- ½ cup artificial sweetener
- 1 cup cranberries
- 1 orange
- 1 cup celery
- ½ cup pecans

## DIRECTIONS

1. In a bowl mix all ingredients and mix well
2. Serve with dressing

Serves: **2**
Prep Time: **5** Minutes
Cook Time: **5** Minutes
Total Time: **10** Minutes

## INGREDIENTS

- 8 oz. romaine lettuce
- 2 cups radicchio
- ¼ red onion
- 2 ribs celery
- 1 cup tomatoes
- 1 can chickpeas
- 1 cup salad dressing

## DIRECTIONS

1. In a bowl mix all ingredients and mix well
2. Serve with dressing

Serves:         *2*
Prep Time:    *5*    Minutes

Cook Time:    *5*    Minutes

Total Time:   *10*   Minutes

## INGREDIENTS

- 2 cans chickpeas
- 2 cups carrots
- 1 cup celery
- ¼ cup green onions
- ¼ cup dill leaves
- ¼ cup olive oil
- 1 cucumber
- 1 cup salad dressing

## DIRECTIONS

1. In a bowl mix all ingredients and mix well
2. Serve with dressing

Serves:        **2**

Prep Time:     **5**   Minutes

Cook Time:     **5**   Minutes

Total Time:    **10**  Minutes

## INGREDIENTS

- 1 cup cooked quinoa
- 1 cup sunflower seeds
- 1 tablespoon olive oil
- 1 head romaine lettuce
- 1 cup carrots
- 1 cup cabbage
- ¼ cup radishes

## DIRECTIONS

1. In a bowl mix all ingredients and mix well
2. Serve with dressing

Serves:        **2**

Prep Time:    **5**    Minutes

Cook Time:    **5**    Minutes

Total Time:   **10**   Minutes

## INGREDIENTS

- 1 bunch coriander leaves
- 1 bunch mint leaves
- ¼ red onion
- 1 bunch parsley
- 1 cup lentils
- 1 tablespoon pumpkin seeds
- 1 tablespoon pine nuts

## DIRECTIONS

1. In a bowl mix all ingredients and mix well
2. Serve with dressing

Serves:        **2**
Prep Time:    **5**  Minutes

Cook Time:    **5**  Minutes

Total Time:  **10**  Minutes

## INGREDIENTS

- 1 cauliflower
- 2 cups cooked quinoa
- 1 can chickpeas
- 1 cup baby spinach
- ¼ cup parsley
- ¼ cup cilantro
- ¼ cup green onion
- ½ cup feta cheese

## DIRECTIONS

1. In a bowl mix all ingredients and mix well
2. Serve with dressing

Serves:          2
Prep Time:      5    Minutes

Cook Time:      5    Minutes

Total Time:    *10*   Minutes

## INGREDIENTS

- 1 head romaine lettuce
- 1 cup tomatoes
- 1 cup cucumber
- 1 cup celery
- ¼ cup olives
- 1 shallot
- 1 cup salad dressing

## DIRECTIONS

1. In a bowl mix all ingredients and mix well
2. Serve with dressing

Serves:          **2**
Prep Time:     **5**   Minutes

Cook Time:    **5**   Minutes

Total Time:   **10**  Minutes

## INGREDIENTS

- 1 cup couscous
- ¼ cup pine nuts
- ¼ cup olive lil
- 1 tablespoon lemon juice
- 1 shallot
- 2 cloves garlic
- 1 tsp salt
- 1 can chickpeas
- 1 cup tomatoes
- ½ cup feta cheese
- 1 zucchini
- 1 tablespoon basil

## DIRECTIONS

1. In a bowl mix all ingredients and mix well
2. Serve with dressing

Serves:        **2**
Prep Time:    **5**    Minutes

Cook Time:   **5**    Minutes

Total Time:   **10**   Minutes

## INGREDIENTS

- 1 cup cooked FARRO
- 1 bay leaf
- 1 shallot
- ¼ cup olive oil
- 2 cups arugula
- ¼ cup parmesan cheese
- ¼ cup basil
- ¼ cup parsley
- ¼ cup pecans

## DIRECTIONS

1. In a bowl mix all ingredients and mix well
2. Serve with dressing

Serves:        2
Prep Time:    5    Minutes
Cook Time:   5    Minutes
Total Time:  10   Minutes

## INGREDIENTS

- 1 head leaf lettuce
- 1 red bell pepper
- 2 mangoes
- ¼ green onion
- ¼ cup peanuts
- ¼ cup cilantro
- 1 cup peanut dressing

## DIRECTIONS

1. In a bowl mix all ingredients and mix well
2. Serve with dressing

## DINNER SALMON

Serves:        **4**
Prep Time:    **10**   Minutes

Cook Time:   **10**   Minutes

Total Time:   **20**   Minutes

### INGREDIENTS

- ½ cup panko breadcrumbs
- 2 cloves garlic
- 2 tbs olive oil
- ¼ tsp black pepper
- 2 tbs parsley
- 1/3 tsp salt
- 1 tsp oregano
- 2 lemons
- 4 salmon fillets

### DIRECTIONS

1. Mix together minced garlic, oregano, chopped parsley, breadcrumbs, zest of 1 lemon, olive oil, and salt

2. Place the salmon fillets on a greased baking sheet and pour the mixture over, tossing the fish well

3. Bake for about 10 minutes

4. Serve topped with lemon juice squeezed over

Serves:          *6*
Prep Time:    *10*   Minutes

Cook Time:    *30*   Minutes

Total Time:   *40*   Minutes

## INGREDIENTS

- 6 chicken thighs
- 1 cup honey
- 1/3 cup ginger
- 1 cup soy sauce
- 1/3 cup garlic

## DIRECTIONS

1. Mix together the soy sauce and honey
2. Stir in the garlic and ginger and mix well to combine
3. Pour the mixture over the chicken and allow to marinate as long as you desire
4. Cook in the preheated oven at 400F for about 20 minutes, then flip over and cook until done

5. Serve with desired vegetables

Serves: **4**

Prep Time: **15** Minutes

Cook Time: **35** Minutes

Total Time: **50** Minutes

## INGREDIENTS

- 2 cutlet racks of lamb
- 4 red onions
- 1 bunch baby carrots
- 5 oz spinach leaves
- 1 ½ lb potatoes
- 4 tbs oil
- Salt
- Pepper

## DIRECTIONS

1. Place the carrots, potatoes, onions and oil into a bowl
2. Season with salt and pepper and toss to combine

3. Place the onions and potatoes into a lined roasting pan

4. Cook for at least 20 minutes

5. Season the racks with salt and pepper and cook in hot oil for about 5 minutes per side until browned

6. Place the lamb and carrots together and cook in the oven for at least 15 minutes

7. Steam the spinach

8. Serve the lamb with the steamed spinach and cooked vegetables

Serves:        *4*

Prep Time:    *10*   Minutes

Cook Time:   *10*   Minutes

Total Time:   *20*   Minutes

## INGREDIENTS

- ½ cup semi-dried tomatoes
- 1/3 cup olives
- 3 tsp olive oil
- 1 ½ cups evaporated milk
- 1 ½ oz spinach
- ¾ lb chicken breast
- 2 green onions
- 1 tbs cornflour
- 1 lb pasta

## DIRECTIONS

1. Cook the pasta

2. Cook the chicken and onion in hot oil until golden

3. Add in the tomatoes and olives

4. Toss well to combine

5. Form a smooth paste by mixing the corn flour and 1 tbs of water

6. Add the mixture to the pan and cook until the sauce thickens

7. Season with salt and pepper

8. Add in the chicken mixture and spinach to pasta

9. Cook for 2 more minutes

10. Serve immediately

Serves:        **6**

Prep Time:    **10**   Minutes

Cook Time:   **30**   Minutes

Total Time:   **40**   Minutes

## INGREDIENTS

- 1 cup breadcrumbs
- 1 cup quinoa
- 8 oz spinach
- Salt
- Pepper

## DIRECTIONS

1. Cook the quinoa
2. Process the spinach using a food processor
3. Mix with the breadcrumbs and cooked quinoa, then season with salt and pepper
4. Form patties form the mixture and bake in the preheated oven at 350F for at least 15 minutes
5. Serve with desired side dishes

Serves: **4**

Prep Time: **5** Minutes

Cook Time: **25** Minutes

Total Time: **30** Minutes

## INGREDIENTS

- 1 cup Sriracha
- 30 oz black beans
- 1 cup corn
- 2 tbs olive oil
- 1 cup water
- 1 red pepper
- 2 tbs chili powder
- 30 oz white beans
- 30 oz kidney beans
- 1 onion
- 5 garlic cloves
- 30 oz tomatoes
- 1 ½ tbs cumin

## DIRECTIONS

1. Peel and mince the garlic
2. Dice the pepper and onion
3. Sauté the onions in olive oil until translucent
4. Add the garlic and pepper
5. Mix in the cumin, Sriracha and chili powder
6. Cook until soft
7. Add the remaining ingredients and allow to simmer for 20 minutes
8. Serve immediately

Serves:          **4**

Prep Time:    **10**   Minutes

Cook Time:   **10**   Minutes

Total Time:   **20**   Minutes

## INGREDIENTS

- 1 cup onion
- 2 cloves garlic
- 3 tbs olive oil
- 8 oz tomato sauce
- 4 cups baby spinach
- 5 cups pasta
- 1/3 cup Kalamata olives
- ½ cup feta cheese
- ¼ cup basil
- 8 oz chicken sausage

## DIRECTIONS

1. Cook the sausage, onion and garlic in hot oil for about 5 minutes
2. Add the tomato sauce, cooked pasta, spinach and olives and cook for 5 minutes
3. Stir in the feta and basil
4. Serve immediately

Serves:          **4**
Prep Time:    **10**   Minutes

Cook Time:    **40**   Minutes

Total Time:    **50**   Minutes

## INGREDIENTS

- 1 lb potatoes
- 1 leek
- 2 shallots
- 3 ¼ oz double cream
- ½ lb chicken
- 2 oz butter
- 3 oz milk
- 1 oz flour
- 1 ¼ cans chicken stock
- 2 ½ oz peas
- 2 tbs parsley
- 2 oz cheese
- 2 tbs lemon juice
- Salt

- Pepper

## DIRECTIONS

1. Cook the potatoes in salted water until tender
2. Drain and mash with milk, butter and grated cheese
3. Cook the shallots and leek in melted butter for 10 minutes
4. Stir in the flour and cook 1 more minute, then slowly pour the stock in to make a sauce
5. Stir in the cream and cook until it comes to the boil
6. Stir in the cooked chicken, parsley and peas, then remove from heat and stir in the lemon juice
7. Season with salt and pepper, then spoon into a dish, topping with the mash
8. Bake in the preheated oven at 400F for about 20 minutes
9. Serve immediately

Serves: **4**

Prep Time: **10** Minutes

Cook Time: **20** Minutes

Total Time: **30** Minutes

## INGREDIENTS

- 4 chicken breasts
- 5 tsp olive oil
- 2 ½ tbs lemon juice
- 5 tbs white wine
- 2 tbs garlic

## DIRECTIONS

1. Cook the chicken and garlic in hot oil until browned on both sides
2. Mix the white wine and lemon juice together
3. Reduce the heat and drizzle the mixture over
4. Cook covered for 15 more minutes
5. Serve immediately

Serves:        **2**
Prep Time:    **10**   Minutes

Cook Time:   **10**   Minutes

Total Time:   **20**   Minutes

## INGREDIENTS

- 2/3 cup barbeque sauce
- 1 1/3 tbs Worcestershire sauce
- 1 ½ tbs butter
- 1 tsp garlic powder
- 1 ½ lb chicken

## DIRECTIONS

1. Melt the butter and stir in the barbeque and Worcestershire sauce, then add the garlic powder
2. Place the chicken into the sauce and coat well
3. Put in a saucepan and simmer covered until cooked through
4. Remove the cover and pour the remaining sauce over, then cook 5 more minutes

## LEMON BARS

Serves: **12**

Prep Time: **10** Minutes

Cook Time: **50** Minutes

Total Time: **60** Minutes

### INGREDIENTS

**Base**
- 2 tbs milk
- 1 ¾ oz rice
- 3 oz sugar
- 6 oz flour
- 5 oz butter

**Topping**
- 7 oz sugar
- ¾ oz flour
- 3 lemons
- 3 eggs

## DIRECTIONS

1. Mix together the sugar, rice and flour with the butter and rub until fine crumbs form

2. Stir in the milk and mix well

3. Press the dough into a prepared tin

4. Bake in the preheated oven at 350F for at least 15 minutes

5. Mix the topping ingredients together and pour over the base

6. Bake for another 10 minutes

7. Allow to cool then serve

# CHOCOLATE PROFITEROLES

Serves:          **6**

Prep Time:    **5**    Minutes

Cook Time:   **10**   Minutes

Total Time:   **15**   Minutes

## INGREDIENTS

- 18 pastry cases
- 1 cup dark chocolate
- 1 cup custard

## DIRECTIONS

1. **Melt the chocolate**
2. **Whisk into the thickened custard**
3. **Refrigerate overnight**
4. **Cut the profiteroles in half**
5. **Spoon the chocolate mixture onto a half, then top with the other one**
6. **Drizzle remaining chocolate over**
7. **Allow to cool, then serve**

Serves: **1**

Prep Time: **5** Minutes

Cook Time: **5** Minutes

Total Time: **10** Minutes

## INGREDIENTS

- ¼ cup chia seeds
- 3 tbs almond butter
- 1 banana
- 1 cup milk
- 3 tbs maple syrup
- 3 tbs walnuts

## DIRECTIONS

1. Mix the chia seeds, maple syrup and milk together
2. Stir well, then refrigerate overnight
3. Add banana, almond butter and walnuts and stir
4. Serve immediately

Serves:        *4*
Prep Time:  *10*  Minutes

Cook Time:  *50*  Minutes

Total Time:  *60*  Minutes

## INGREDIENTS

- 1 cup pumpkin puree
- 1/3 tsp sea salt
- 2 tbs vanilla
- 1/3 cup coconut palm sugar
- 1 ½ cup milk
- 1/3 tsp pumpkin spice
- 2 eggs
- 3 tbs cornstarch
- 1 tsp cinnamon

## DIRECTIONS

1. Mix the pumpkin puree, milk, eggs and vanilla

2. Separately, mix spices, sea salt, cornstarch and coconut sugar together

3. Sift the sugar mixture into the pumpkin mixture and mix well

4. Pour into cups then place the cups into a baking pan

5. Add water to come halfway up the sides of the cups

6. Bake for about 50 minutes in the preheated oven at 350F

7. Allow to cool, then serve

Serves:        *1*
Prep Time:    *2*   Minutes

Cook Time:   *3*   Minutes

Total Time:   *5*   Minutes

## INGREDIENTS

- Berries
- 5 tbs yogurt
- Honey

## DIRECTIONS

1. Pour 2 tbs of yogurt in a jar
2. Drizzle some honey, then top with the berries
3. Repeat until the jar is full
4. Serve immediately

Serves: **4**

Prep Time: **10** Minutes

Cook Time: **50** Minutes

Total Time: **60** Minutes

### INGREDIENTS
Crust
- 2 cups rolled oats
- 12 medjool dates

Filling
- 3 tsp agar-agar
- 2 1/3 cups mixed berries
- 4 mandarins
- 4 ½ cups yogurt

### DIRECTIONS

1. Place the crust ingredients together in a food processor, add a pinch of salt and process until finely chopped
2. While still running, pour some water until the mixture sticks together

3. Press the mixture into a baking pan
4. Mix the agar-agar with water and bring to a boil, then allow to boil for 5 minutes
5. Puree the berries and mix with the yogurt, then heat a little bit
6. Stir the agar-agar mixture into the yogurt
7. Pour the mixture over the crust and top with mandarin slices
8. Allow to refrigerate for at least 1 hour
9. Serve when ready

Serves: **6**

Prep Time: **10** Minutes

Cook Time: **15** Minutes

Total Time: **25** Minutes

## INGREDIENTS

- 3 cups strawberries
- Sugar
- Whipped topping
- 15 oz pie crust
- 2 cups yogurt

## DIRECTIONS

1. Cut the crust into circles
2. Press the dough into a muffin pan, then place another muffin pan into the filled one to shape the dough while baking
3. Bake for about 10 minutes until golden
4. Fill with yogurt and strawberries, then top with whipped cream and sugar

Serves:          **6**

Prep Time:    **5**    Minutes

Cook Time:   **10**   Minutes

Total Time:   **15**   Minutes

## INGREDIENTS

- 3 tsp vanilla
- 1 cup granulated sugar
- ½ cup cocoa powder
- ¼ cup cornstarch
- 2 1/3 cups milk
- 3 tbs butter
- ¼ tsp salt

## DIRECTIONS

1. Mix cocoa, sugar, salt and cornstarch in a pot
2. Slowly pour the milk in while whisking
3. Set pot over heat and stir continuously for about 8 minutes, then reduce the heat and stir for 1 more minute

4. Remove from heat and stir in butter and vanilla

5. Pour into bowls, allow to cool, then refrigerate until firm

6. Serve cold

Serves:        **16**

Prep Time:   **10**   Minutes

Cook Time:   **80**   Minutes

Total Time:  **90**   Minutes

## INGREDIENTS

- 1 egg
- 1 cup stale bread
- ¼ cup cranberries
- 2/3 cup milk
- ¼ cup raisins
- 1 1/3 cup water
- 2/3 cup brown sugar
- ¼ tsp mixed spices

## DIRECTIONS

1. Put the bread into a bowl and pour the water over
2. Allow to soak for 1 hour

3. Drain the water from bread and squeeze the excess out

4. Mix the bread with the remaining ingredients and place into a greased baking tin

5. Cook for about 80 minutes until golden brown

6. Allow to cool, then cut into squares

7. Serve cold

# AVOCADO PUDDING

Serves:        **2**

Prep Time:     **5**    Minutes

Cook Time:     **5**    Minutes

Total Time:    **10**   Minutes

## INGREDIENTS

- ½ avocado
- 1 ½ tbs cocoa powder
- 1 banana
- Maple syrup

## DIRECTIONS

1. Blend the ingredients together until smooth using a food processor
2. Add some maple syrup and stir again
3. Allow to chill in the refrigerator
4. Serve cold

## OMBRE SMOOTHIE

Serves:        *1*

Prep Time:    *5*   Minutes

Cook Time:   *5*   Minutes

Total Time:   *10*   Minutes

### INGREDIENTS

- 1 pineapple
- 1 mango
- 1 cup water
- 1 cup raspberries

### DIRECTIONS

1. **In a blender place all ingredients and blend until smooth**
2. **Pour smoothie in a glass and serve**

# TURMERIC SMOOTHIE

Serves:        *1*
Prep Time:     5   Minutes
Cook Time:     5   Minutes
Total Time:    *10*   Minutes

## INGREDIENTS

- 2 cups mango
- 1 cup Greek Yogurt
- ¼ cup orange juice
- 1 banana
- 1 tablespoon turmeric
- 1 tablespoon agave nectar
- 1 cup ice
- ¼ tsp vanilla extract

## DIRECTIONS

1. In a blender place all ingredients and blend until smooth
2. Pour smoothie in a glass and serve

Serves:          *1*
Prep Time:    5    Minutes

Cook Time:    5    Minutes

Total Time:   *10*   Minutes

## INGREDIENTS

- 1 pinch cinnamon
- 1 cup raspberries
- 1 cup almond milk
- 2 dates
- 1 cup ice

## DIRECTIONS

1. **In a blender place all ingredients and blend until smooth**
2. **Pour smoothie in a glass and serve**

# BERRIES SMOOTHIE

Serves:        *1*
Prep Time:    5    Minutes
Cook Time:   5    Minutes
Total Time:  *10*   Minutes

## INGREDIENTS

- 1 cup berries
- 1 banana
- ½ cup orange juice
- 1 cup ice

## DIRECTIONS

1. In a blender place all ingredients and blend until smooth
2. Pour smoothie in a glass and serve

# MACA SMOOTHIE

Serves:          *1*

Prep Time:    *5*   Minutes

Cook Time:   *5*   Minutes

Total Time:   *10*   Minutes

## INGREDIENTS

- 2 cups hemp link
- 1 cup ice
- ¼ cup lemon juice
- 2 mangoes
- 2 oz. mango juice
- ½ tablespoon maca powder
- 1 tsp vanilla extract
- 1 tablespoon flaxseeds

## DIRECTIONS

1. **In a blender place all ingredients and blend until smooth**
2. **Pour smoothie in a glass and serve**

# BERRY SMOOTHIE

| | |
|---|---|
| Serves: | *1* |
| Prep Time: | *5* Minutes |
| Cook Time: | *5* Minutes |
| Total Time: | *10* Minutes |

## INGREDIENTS

- 1 cup cherry juice
- 1 cup baby spinach
- 1 cup Greek Yogurt
- 1 avocado
- 1 cup berries
- 1 tablespoon chia seeds

## DIRECTIONS

1. In a blender place all ingredients and blend until smooth
2. Pour smoothie in a glass and serve

Serves:        *1*
Prep Time:    *5*   Minutes

Cook Time:    *5*   Minutes

Total Time:   *10*  Minutes

## INGREDIENTS

- 2 cups peaches
- 1 cup apricots
- 1 banana
- 1 cup milk
- 1 tsp vanilla extract
- 1 tablespoon mint
- 1 cup ice
- Mint leaves

## DIRECTIONS

1. **In a blender place all ingredients and blend until smooth**
2. **Pour smoothie in a glass and serve**

Serves:          *1*
Prep Time:    **5**    Minutes

Cook Time:    **5**    Minutes

Total Time:   ***10***   Minutes

## INGREDIENTS

- 1 cup coconut milk
- ¼ cup orange juice
- 1 banana
- 1 cup mango juice
- ¼ cup Greek yogurt
- 1 tsp lemon juice

## DIRECTIONS

1. **In a blender place all ingredients and blend until smooth**
2. **Pour smoothie in a glass and serve**

Serves:        **1**

Prep Time:    **5**    Minutes

Cook Time:    **5**    Minutes

Total Time:    **10**    Minutes

## INGREDIENTS

- **4 strawberries**
- **½ cup watermelon**
- **½ cup peaches**
- **2 scoops raspberries**
- **2 oz. orange juice**

## DIRECTIONS

1. **In a blender place all ingredients and blend until smooth**
2. **Pour smoothie in a glass and serve**

# KALE-GINGER SMOOTHIE

Serves:           *1*

Prep Time:     **5**    Minutes

Cook Time:    **5**    Minutes

Total Time:    **10**   Minutes

## INGREDIENTS

- 1 cup kale
- 1 banana
- 1 cup almond milk
- 1 tsp chia seeds
- ½ avocado
- 1 tsp ginger
- 1 cup ice

## DIRECTIONS

1. **In a blender place all ingredients and blend until smooth**
2. **Pour smoothie in a glass and serve**

# THANK YOU FOR READING THIS BOOK!

Printed in Great Britain
by Amazon

35477374R00061